The 5:2 Diet:

Uncover The Secret to Losing Weight While Living A Healthier, Happier Life!

Kevin Hughes © 2017

Disclaimer:

This book is for informational purposes only and the author, his agents, heirs, and assignees do not accept any responsibilities for any liabilities, actual or alleged, resulting from the use of this information.

This report is not "professional advice." The author encourages the reader to seek advice from a professional where any reasonably prudent person would do so. While every reasonable attempt has been made to verify the information contained in this eBook, the author and his affiliates cannot assume any responsibility for errors, inaccuracies or omissions, including omissions in transmission or reproduction.

Any references to people, events, organizations, or business entities are for educational and illustrative purposes only, and no intent to falsely characterize, recommend, disparage, or injure is intended or should be so construed. Any results stated or implied are consistent with general results, but this means results can and will vary. The author, his agents, and assigns, make no promises or guarantees, stated or implied. Individual results will vary and this work is supplied strictly on an "at your own risk" basis.

Introduction

Thanks for grabbing my book "The 5:2 Diet: Uncover The Secret to Losing Weight While Living A Healthier, Happier Life!!" By reading this guide you've decided that you're interested in uncovering all the benefits that the 5:2 diet can have on improving your health and overall well-being. I'm not going to lie and say this is the easiest path to go down. It's not! It will take both hard work and dedication on your part to achieve your goals, especially in the beginning stages. However, after a slight readjustment period, you'll begin to feel lighter and healthier than you have in years.

This book will teach you everything you need to know to begin correctly following a 5:2 diet. I'll be going through the entire process and how you can fast both safely and effectively. I've also included a full resource guide with links to tools, apps, resources, and books to help you along on your journey. If that's not enough I've also packed this guide with over 50+ healthy low-calorie meals to get you going in the right direction.

I'm excited to get started. Let's begin!

Chapter One: The 5:2 Diet Basics

What Is The 5:2 Diet?

The 5:2 diet, also known as The Fast Diet, is an extremely popular form of intermittent fasting. It was popularized back in 2012, by a British journalist and doctor named Michael Mosley. He put forth the idea that one should try eating a normal healthy diet 5 days of the week and fast on the other 2 days restricting one's caloric intake to between 500 and 600 calories per day. This type of fasting regimen is more of an eating pattern than an actual diet. There are no requirements on what foods you're allowed to consume. Instead, the requirements fall around when you're allowed to eat them. I will state that one should still stick to a sensible diet if they want to get the best results out of this diet. If you decide to gorge yourself on your non-fasting days you won't get the benefits of fasting.

How to Get Going On The 5:2 Diet

The 5:2 diet is quite simple to begin. Pick which days you'll be fasting on and what days you'll be eating normally. I suggest sticking to around 2000 to 2400 calories on your non-fasting days depending on your set of caloric needs. This number would be lower for most women at around 1800 calories. Your fasting days need to be split apart. Do not fast 2 days in a row. On fasting days I tend to eat 2 small meals and 1 snack. On my non-fasting days, I eat 3 slightly bigger meals and 1 snack. I find this balance allows me to transition easily from my fasting to non-fasting days. This is the eating schedule that I found works best for me. Feel free to play around with your eating schedule until you find one that works for you.

In the next chapter, I give a bunch of sample daily meal plans you can follow to get started quickly. Whether you follow them or not is up to your discretion. I would recommend that you try planning out your meals each week in advance. This is a smart idea for one main reason. It will allow you to still eat healthy on days when you're tired or feeling rushed to make a meal. Having all your ingredients on hand will cut down on the amount of time needed to make your meals and will also save you unnecessary trips to the store. When I first got started I didn't follow this advice. It led to me having to restart my diet on numerous occasions after cheating. Not being prepared in advance threw me into a downward spiral when I had low energy levels and didn't have ingredients conveniently on hand. Once I started stacking the odds in my favor, success came more naturally.

Is It Healthy?

Fasting short term is not for everyone. For instance, children, pregnant woman, and people with certain medical condition should probably avoid intermittent fasting. For the rest of us, short-term fasting provides no risk to our overall health or well-being. In fact, there have been a lot of studies in recent years that show intermittent fasting such as the 5:2 diet actually provide us with an enormous amount of health benefits. A few of these health benefits include weight loss, reduced insulin levels, lower blood sugar levels, improved insulin sensitivity, heart arrhythmias, allergies, asthma, and hot flashes.

From a dieting perspective, intermittent fasting has been shown to improve a person's odds of sticking to a diet over regular forms of dieting. People have more issues sticking to a diet involving continuous restriction of calories over a diet designed to only restrict your caloric intake during certain designated periods of time.

During one study that lasted 3 months and split people into a fasting group and non-fasting group, the fasting group had reduced their weight by more than 10 pounds more than the regular dieting non-fasting group. On top of that, they had reduced their overall fast mass by more than 7 pounds with no changes in their muscles mass over the non-fasting group. They also decreased their triglyceride levels by 20%, their leptin levels by 40% and reduced their levels of CRP which is a crucial marker of inflammation in our bodies.

If you want to get the most out of your 5:2 diet you should pair it with an exercise program. I went with an endurance program, while I have many friends who stick to weight training or a combination of the two. No matter what form of exercise plan you choose it's important to choose something even if you only do it a few times per week. I started myself off slow and went from exercising 2 days a week to now at least 4 days if not 5 days each week depending on my schedule.

Eating On Fasting Days

I often get asked the questions "How should I eat on fasting days?" and "What should I eat on fasting days?"

Here are my answers to both:

There is no rule as to what or when you need to eat during your fasting days. Everyone has a different schedule and pattern that they prefer. That being said, there are some general guidelines I'd like to share that most people tend to stick to.

1. There are two different eating patterns the majority of people fall into. The first is eating 3 times a day. These are either 3 small meals or 2 meals and 1 smaller snack. The other popular method is only eating 2 times each day, those meals usually being lunch and dinner.

2. Since you're only allowed a limited amount of calories on your fasting days you need to budget them wisely. Spread your meals out during the day. Try not to group them to close together or when you get hungry later in the day you'll either want to cheat on your diet or spend the rest of your day feeling hungry and upset.

3. Focus on including nutritious, high protein, high fiber foods that will leave you feeling full even though you haven't consumed a ton of calories.

4. Soups are a wonderful option during your fast days. There have been a lot of studies that show soups leave a person feeling fuller for a longer period of time than if you had the same types of foods in their original form. I have a variety of soups I enjoy that can be rotated in and out of my meal plans each week so I never get bored with what I'm having.

Fasting Days Allowable Food Examples:

Vegetables

Lean Meat

Grilled Fish

Soups (Miso, Vegetable, Cauliflower, or Tomato)

Baked or Boiled Eggs

Cauliflower Rice

Natural Yogurt w/ Berries

Water

Black Coffee

Tea

What to Do If You Still Feel Hungry or Feeling Weaker Than Normal

During the initial part of the 5:2 diet, you can expect at times to feel overwhelmingly hungry while on your fasting days. During this period it's also completely normal to feel a little slower, foggier, or weaker than you normally would. This is your body adjusting to your new eating pattern and flushing out some of the harmful toxins that have built up in your system from years of poor eating habits. I found that within a few weeks you should not only be back to normal but actually feeling an improvement over how you felt when starting out.

You'll be shocked at how quickly the feeling of hunger begins to fade away. I found the beginning fasts to be quite challenging but I soon noticed that my fasting days had become easier and easier until I barely gave it a thought anymore. To be safe I suggest always keeping a small snack on hand during the initial fasting periods in case you begin to feel ill or extremely weak. If you do begin to feel ill or weak, especially on multiple occasions, I would suggest to stop fasting until you spoke with your physician and made sure it was safe for you to continue.

Who Should Avoid Trying The 5:2 Diet?

Although intermittent fasting has been shown to be safe for healthier, well-nourished people, it does not mean that it's right for everyone.

Some people have to avoid restrictive diets and any kind of fasting:

Nursing mothers, children, teenagers, pregnant women, and individuals suffering from type 1 diabetes.

Women who are trying to get pregnant or have had issues with their fertility.

People that are underweight or malnourished.

Individuals that are sensitive to drops in their blood sugar levels.

Individuals that have a history of prior eating disorders.

Women, in general, tend to benefit less from intermittent fasting than men.

The 5:2 Diet Frequently Asked Questions

Here are answers to a few common 5:2 diet questions.

1. Will fasting on a 5:2 diet slow down my metabolism?

No. Many studies have come to the conclusion that shorter-term fasts, such as those found in the 5:2 diet only help to boost metabolism. On the other side, fasts lasting longer than 3 days can help to slow down your metabolism. These type of lengthier fasts are not part of a 5:2 diet and will therefore not be an issue to anyone following this type of diet.

2. Can I skip breakfast? I thought it was the most important meal of the day?

Yes, you can absolutely skip breakfast while fasting. Skipping meals while fasting has been shown to have a positive effect as long as you maintain an overall balanced and healthy diet.

3. Are liquids allowed during the 5:2 diet fasting days?

Yes. You're allowed to drink coffee, tea, water, and other non-caloric beverages. What you're not allowed to do is add any sugar to your coffee. A small amount of milk or cream is acceptable. Coffee is a popular drink among people on the 5:2 diet as it helps to blunt one's hunger when fasting.

4. I cheated on my 5:2 diet. What do I do now?

The simple answer is to forget about your past slip and get back onto the diet. For example, if you ended up cheating by consuming more than 600 calories on your fasting day, then consider this one of your normal days and try to fast on the next day or add another day during your week that better suits your schedule. Remember, the 5:2 diet only requires you to fast 2 days each week. It doesn't specify what 2 days those need to be. Don't give up because you think you failed or cheated. I always schedule my fasting days for the earlier part of the week that way in case I slip up I still have a few days to make up the lost fasting day without getting too far off course.

5. Can I exercise during fasting days to earn more calories?

You can exercise on your fasting days. However, since your calorie intake is lower on these days you should stick to a less vigorous workout. You can never buy calories. Any exercise you do on these days is just a bonus to your weight loss and health. You can't exercise on these days to earn more food.

6. Are supplements allowed on fasting days?

Yes. However, remember various supplements such as fat-soluble vitamins will work better when taken with meals.

7. Will fasting days on the 5:2 diet cause any muscle loss?

It might. Every sort of weight loss method can lead to someone losing muscle. That is why it's crucial that your exercise routine contains weight lifting exercises. You should also take in a higher amount of protein. Studies have taught us that a 5:2 diet causes less muscle loss than if you were restricting your caloric intake as you would during a conventional diet.

8. What foods should I have on fasting days?

While there aren't any restrictions as to the types of foods you can eat while following this diet there are some guidelines I would suggest sticking to in order to optimize your results. Remember you want to stay between 500 to 600 calories on your 2 fasting days.

Foods to Avoid:

Fried foods (frying foods often leads to higher calorie counts than if you had prepared the same food using a different method).

Processed or refined carbohydrates such as pasta, bread, rice, canned vegetables, and sugary sweets.

Salad dressings and sauces (A huge source of empty calories).

Fruit drinks, alcoholic beverages, soda, and drinks containing artificial sweeteners.

<u>Foods to Try Instead:</u>

Small-sized portions of fish or lean meat.

Whole grains (the increased fiber helps to boost metabolism and helps to lower blood sugar, cholesterol, and weight.)

Fresh vegetables and fruits.

Coffee and tea.

Plenty of water.

What Steps Can I Take If I'm Not Losing Weight?

There are a few simple reasons why you might not be losing the weight as expected.

1. Your caloric intake on your fasting days is over the 500 to 600 calorie mark.

2. You've been consuming too many calories on your non-fasting days.

Always keep an eye out for hidden calories. You might not even realize you're cheating on your diet. At first, I had trouble losing the weight and it wasn't until I went over everything I consumed with a fine tooth comb that I realized I was taking in too many calories from juices and energy drinks. I thought I was cutting back by cutting out soda but I didn't realize the number of calories most juices contained in them. Once I figured out what I was doing wrong I was able to make the correct adjustments and the weight began to fall off.

Remember, weight loss on the scale isn't everything. After a few weeks, the weight loss will begin to slow down. However, your body is continuing to transform due to the increase in muscle mass, which weighs more than fat does in your body. Weight can fluctuate due to fluids in your body and hormones. Don't weigh yourself every day or get too obsessed with the numbers on the scale. I find weighing yourself once a week is more than enough. I also suggest to measure yourself once every month around your hips, waist, legs, and arms. This will allow you to see how your body is truly beginning to transform over time. I find it to be a great indicator of my overall progress.

If for some reason you're still having trouble losing weight even after cleaning up your diet, I suggest adding more exercise to your weekly routine. I suggest getting yourself a pedometer so you can track all your steps each day. A good goal to strive for is 10,000 steps a day.

Chapter Two: The 5:2 Diet Recipe Meal Plan Options

In this chapter, I'll be discussing different 5:2 diet recipe meal plan options on both fasting and non-fasting days. Both sets of days are equally important because if you stray off course during one set of days you'll negatively affect the results you're able to achieve. If you slip don't get too down on yourself. Just get back onto the diet and continue forward. If you find you're struggling during certain points try mixing things up. You can do this by either changing up the times of the days you eat, the days that choose to fast on or by the types of meals that you're preparing for yourself. Personally, it took some experimentation with my meal times and what types of meals before settling into a comfortable groove. Don't get discouraged. You'll eventually begin to find a routine that works for you and your lifestyle.

I haven't included any drinks with these meal plans. You're allowed to drink coffee, teas, water, and other non-caloric beverages on your fasting days. I would also try to follow the same advice on non-fast days but that would be up to you. I've always found it was easier to stick to non-caloric beverages all the time instead of going back and forth. Try avoiding any drinks with a high sugar content in them. That includes regular soda and most juices.

5:2 Diet Fasting Day Meal Plans

Following a 5:2 diet can be difficult at first. It's a big change to our way of eating to fast multiple days each week. In order to make this process a bit smoother, I've dedicated this section to quick and simple 5:2 diet recipe plans for the days that you're fasting on. These meals are all right around the 500 calorie mark. I think these meal options do a good job at leaving you feeling full while also giving you the nutrients you need. I find that planning out my meals in advance each week takes a lot of the pressure off of me. The last thing you need when fasting is additional stress on your body.

These meal plans are only suggestions. Feel free to take from them what you like and discard what you don't. I hope they'll give you an idea of the types of daily meal plans you'll want to put together for yourself going forward. Don't be afraid to spice things up a little bit through the use of seasonings and other herbs. Just be sure they don't contain any additional calories. For example, I love adding a squeeze of lemon to my salads and seasoning certain meals with cracked black pepper.

Fasting Plan #1

Breakfast: 3 1/2 ounces of Low-Fat Natural Yogurt & Sweet Plums - 145 calories

Dinner: 2 Ryvita Crisp Bread Crackers & 2 ounces of Tuna - 250 calories

Snack: Miso Soup - 30 calories

Total Calorie Count: 425 calories

Fasting Plan #2

Breakfast: 1 1/2 ounce sachet of Quaker Oats Porridge - 250 calories

Dinner: Feta, Spinach, & Beetroot Salad (1 ounce of Feta, 2 ounces of Spinach, & 1 3/4 ounces of Beetroot) - 125 calories

Snack: Apple Slices w/ 1 tablespoon of Almond Butter - 145 calories

Total Calorie Count: 520 calories

Fasting Plan #3

Breakfast: Belvita Breakfast Biscuits - 225 calories

Dinner: Roasted Vegetables (1/2 red pepper, 1/2 butternut squash, 1/2 aubergine, 1/2 zucchini.) w/ 1 tablespoon of Balsamic Glaze - 260 calories

Snack: Jell-O Sugar-Free Low-Calorie Jello - 10 calories

Total Calorie Count: 495

Fasting Plan #4

Breakfast: 1 Soft Boiled Egg & 5 pieces of Asparagus - 90 calories

Dinner: Turkey Burgers w/ 1 Corn-On-The-Cob - 350 calories

Snack: A Handful of Grapes - 80 calories

Total Calorie Count: 520 calories

Fasting Plan #5

Breakfast: 1 Banana and 3 1/2 ounces of Low-Fat Yogurt - 175 calories

Dinner: 4 1/2 ounce Turkey Breast w/ 1 cup of Cooked Wilted Spinach - 215 calories

Snack: 1/2 ounce of Popcorn - 70 calories

Total Calorie Count: 460

Fasting Plan #6

Breakfast: Spinach Omelette (2 Eggs & 2 ounces of Spinach Leaves) - 160 calories

Dinner: 1 1/2 ounces of Hummus & Medium Bowl of Cucumber, Carrots, & Green Pepper - 175 calories

Snack: 2 ounces of Edamame Beans & Rock Salt - 85 calories

Total Calorie Count: 420

Fasting Plan #7

Breakfast: Mixed Berry Bowl (3 1/2 ounces of Raspberries, Strawberries, & Blueberries) - 115 calories

Dinner: 4 1/2 ounces of Harissa Chicken w/ 3 1/2 ounces of Chargrilled Vegetable Couscous - 315 calories

Snack: 10 Pistachios - 60 calories

Total Calorie Count - 490 calories

Fasting Plan #8

Breakfast: 1 Apple, 1 Carrot & Ginger Smoothie - 110 calories

Dinner: Pitta Pizza - 250 calories

Snack: 5 ounces of Blueberries - 140 calories

Total Calorie Count: 500 calories

Fasting Plan #9

Breakfast: 1 1/2 ounces of Fruit & Nut Muesli - 200 calories

Dinner: 3 1/2 ounce Salmon (w/ 3 teaspoons of Green Pesto) & 3 1/2 ounces of Steamed Kale - 300 calories

Snack: 2 ounces of Cherries - 25 calories

Total Calorie Count: 525 calories

Fasting Plan #10

Breakfast: 3 Weight Watchers Blueberry Buttermilk Pancakes - 190 calories

Dinner: 6-ounce Halibut Fillet w/ 1 cup of Sugar Snap Peas - 275 calories

Snack: 1 tablespoon of Sunflower & Pumpkin Seeds- 90 calories

Total Calorie Count: 555 calories

5:2 Diet Non-Fasting Day Meal Plans

I've found that many people starting a 5:2 diet end up having the most difficulty sticking to a sensible diet on their non-fasting days. Since there are no specific diet restrictions one needs to follow on these days many people will often overindulge or eat the wrong kinds of foods. Remember, if you want the diet to work you need to pay as much attention to your meals on non-fasting days as you do on your fasting days. Here are some easy to follow daily meal plans to help you get started in the right direction. Feel free to make any substitutions you like. This is just a guideline to show you the types of meals you should be making for yourself.

During my non-fasting days, I'm not worried about counting my calories. The reason for this is I know I'm only eating 3 sensible meals and 1 snack during my day. This allows me to plan my meals out in advance so on days that I'm tired or in a hurry I don't cave in and pig out on fast food or other quick unhealthy options. During the first few weeks on this diet, I allow myself a few more carbs than I will going forward. Eventually, I suggest trying to cut out most cakes and bread altogether.

Non-Fasting Plan #1

Breakfast: 7 ounces of Greek Style Yogurt w/ 3 1/2 ounces of Mixed Berries (Raspberries, Strawberries, & Blueberries)

Lunch: Mixed Assortment of Sushi (Your Preference) & Miso Soup

Dinner: Tofu & Asian Vegetable Stir Fry w/ Ginger & Garlic Sauce

Snack: 1 bag of Popcorn

<u>Non-Fasting Plan #2</u>

Breakfast: 2 Egg Omelette w/ 1 Piece of Toast

Lunch: Chicken Caesar Salad w/ Light Dressing

Dinner: 6 ounces of Fillet Steak w/ Baked Potato & Beans

Snack: 4 ounces of Unsweetened Applesauce Sprinkled w/ Cinnamon

<u>Non-Fasting Plan #3</u>

Breakfast: Crumbled Feta w/ 1/2 an Avocado & Lime Juice On Toasted Rye

Lunch: 15 ounces of Chicken & Vegetable Soup w/ 2 Crackers

Dinner: Grilled Sea Bass w/ Roasted Root Vegetables

Snack: 8 Grape Tomatoes Dipped In 1 tablespoon of Light Cream Cheese

<u>Non-Fasting Plan #4</u>

Breakfast: 2 slices of Honey Roast Ham w/ 2 Poached Eggs

Lunch: Poached Salmon w/ Small Potato Salad & Mixed Leaf Salad

Dinner: Small Grilled Chicken Breast (Skin Removed) w/ 3 1/2 ounces of Salad w/ Light Dressing

Snack: 1 Apple w/ Soy Butter

<u>*Non-Fasting Plan #5*</u>

Breakfast: Medium Bowl of Porridge w/ 1 tablespoon of Blanched Almonds & 1 Grated Apple

Lunch: 1 bowl of Chili w/ 2 Crackers

Dinner: 5 Stir-Fried King Prawns w/ Grated Ginger & Brown Rice Noodles

Snack: 1 cup of Strawberries w/ 1 Small Low-Fat Yogurt

Chapter Three: 20+ 5:2 Diet Tips & Tricks

1. This one is a no-brainer. Drink a lot of water. A great rule is 64 ounces or 8 cups a day.

2. When starting a fasting day stay busy with meaningful work. I tend to get my best work done while I'm on an empty stomach.

3. Have a lot of protein in each meal. More protein leads to better appetite control and will help to burn fat and build muscle.

4. Drink tea and coffee to help keep your appetite in check. Caffeine is a known natural appetite suppressant. Avoid drinking about 10 hours before you go to bed.

5. Get your most productive work done during the morning. This will help keep your mind occupied and off of food.

6. Workout with weights. There is less point of fasting if you don't plan to workout using weights. You need to build your muscle mass to take full advantage of all the benefits that come from the 5:2 diet.

7. Make the diet flexible for you. Creating your own schedule allows you to have the 5:2 diet work for you instead of you being a slave to it. This diet plan was meant to give you options.

8. Play around with the "timing" of your eating schedule. It's important to follow a structured program for the first 2 to 3 weeks before going off and experimenting on your own. You need to follow a structured program at first and then you can play around with your fasting times and determine what schedule best suits your needs.

9. Stick to this diet for at least 3 weeks before making a final determination on if this diet is right for you. Your body needs this time to adapt.

10. Don't use the non-fasting days as a reason to eat a bunch of bad food. All calories are not created equally. 100 calories of chocolate are not the same as 100 calories of vegetables. When you find yourself about to cheat take a couple minutes and think through what you're doing. Eat whole foods and keep carbs to your post-workout window. Fill up with vegetables and include plenty of protein in each meal.

11. Live life to the fullest. Go crazy when you want. This diet is all about lifestyle and freedom. Just understand you'll need to adjust your calorie intake during the following day or two.

12. Take Vitamin B. It helps you cope with stress and maintain healthy energy levels.

13. Integrate this diet into your daily lifestyle. Begin by slowly delaying breakfast. Doing this will allow you to ease it into your life until you get to a time you can live with. My time is about 1 pm.

14. Don't announce to other people that you're currently fasting. Even though this diet is beginning to gain more mainstream recognition, there are still a ton of folks who don't get the benefits of the 5:2 diet. You don't need additional pressure or negativity putting you in the wrong mindset.

15. Exercise but don't feel the need to overdo it. I recommend combining an exercise routine with your 5:2 diet to see the optimal results. That being said, I know many who burn themselves out by hitting their workouts too hard. These people tend to give up on the diet altogether or struggle to eat healthily.

16. Drink water when you get up in the morning. Often when we feel hungry in the morning, it's because we haven't had a drink of water for the past 8 hours. A healthy weight loss habit to follow is to drink 2 cups of water shortly after waking up.

17. Your first meal will set the tone for your remaining meals that day. Keep your first meal each day as healthy as you can because it will keep you on track for your following meals. This tip made sticking to my diet a breeze. Conversely, whenever I ate poorly during my initial daily meal I continued to struggle throughout the rest of the day. Set yourself up for success from the get-go.

18. Consider where the source of your hunger stems from. A feeling of hunger is often brought on by other outside stimuli that don't include actual hunger. Some examples include, stress, dehydration, anxiety, and feelings of sadness. Once you've determined the reason you're hungry you'll be better equipped to deal with that hunger.

19. Don't sit around your house. There is way too much temptation waiting for you at home. Get creative and do something active while fasting.

20. Understand what else is happening in your life at the time. The 5:2 diet is an eating pattern that will work. However, it only "works" when it's part of your daily routine. The 5:2 diet shouldn't feel like an obligation or a punishment. If this type of diet is doing more harm than good to your psychological well-being, it might not be right for you. The whole point is to get healthier and decrease stress levels.

21. When fasting stay busy with meaningful work. I tend to get my best work done while I'm on an empty stomach.

22. Know yourself. Observe your personal experiences carefully. When it comes to your well-being pretend you're a scientist. Begin the 5:2 diet, gather new data, gain insights, and come up with conclusions that you can use to help decide future action. Always do what's best for you.

23. Respect the cues your body gives you. Paying attention to these cues is extremely important. These cues can include big changes in your appetite and hunger including food cravings, energy levels, sleep quality, mood control, athletic performance, emotional health, physical health, and appearance.

24. Expect there to be peaks and valleys. They are a normal part of life. By keeping an open mind and not freaking out during "down" periods you'll figure out how to have more "ups."

Chapter Four: The 5:2 Diet Resources, Apps, & Books

The 5:2 Diet Resource Guide

In this section, I will go over my top 5:2 diet resources. If you have any additional questions these resources should be able to help.

Recipe Calorie Counter - When you want to count your calories. Just type in your recipe and it spits out all the nutrition information. It's quick and it's free.

https://www.verywell.com/recipe-nutrition-analyzer-4129594

The 5:2 Diet Forums - A good place for sharing your story, staying motivated on your diet, and answering any questions you might have from people who have been through it.

https://thefastdiet.co.uk/forums/

The 5:2 Diet Website - Learn more about how to get started. A good variety of helpful tools to help you in your journey.

https://thefastdiet.co.uk/

The 5:2 Diet App Guide

In this section, I'm going to go over all my favorite apps related to the 5:2 diet. These are all apps that I've used at least once before. I may have missed some but this section will help give you an idea of the variety of apps that are available. I suggest trying a couple out and keeping those that fit your needs.

5:2 Fast Diet Desserts - Free app available only on the iOS. A collection of tasty dessert options w/ calorie amounts included.

5:2 Fast Diet Tracker - Free app available only on Android. Great app specific to people following a 5:2 fast. Lots of helpful features and tracking.

5:2 Fasting Diet Recipes - Available only on the iOS. Costs $1.99. Has 80+ recipes separated by calories amounts.

Fasting Secret - Available only on the iOS. The basic version is free but it also offers a $1.99 upgrade. Works well with the 5:2 diet.

Intermittent Fasting - Free app available on the Android. A robust set of features. Easy to use.

MyFitnessPal - Free app available on both **Android** and iOS. Great set of features for tracking any diet. Excellent set of features.

The 5:2 Diet Book Guide

Here are some of my favorite books on the 5:2 diet. I've read a few books over the years on this subject and these are a few of the ones that left the biggest impression.

1. **The FastDiet** by Michael Mosley

2. **The 5:2 Diet (Feast for 5 Days, Fast for 2)** by Kate Harrison

3. **The Complete Guide to Fasting** by Jason Fung

Chapter Five: The 5:2 Diet Breakfast Recipes

In this chapter, I will share with you 15+ 5:2 diet breakfast recipes you can easily make yourself. I'll include a few beginner recipes and a few recipes that are more advanced. These recipes are all under 600 calories per serving and will work on both your fasting days and non-fasting days. On fasting days you may want to stick to a 1/2 serving for each of your two meals otherwise you'll exceed your calorie allowance for the day.

Vegetable Omelette with Salsa (Serves 2)

Ingredients:

Omelette:

2 cups of 1% Milk or Skim Milk

4 Eggs

Salt

Pepper

Filling:

3 1/2 ounces of Whole Cherry Tomatoes

2 3/4 ounces of Fine Asparagus Spears

3 1/2 ounces of Baby Corn

3 1/2 ounces of Thickly Sliced Mushrooms

Serve:

3 1/2 ounces of Fresh Salsa

Directions:

1. Beat the eggs with your milk, and season with your pepper and salt.

2. Slice your baby sweetcorn in half and add along with your asparagus to a large-sized frying pan. Saute for around 5 minutes.

3. Add your thickly sliced mushrooms and whole cherry tomatoes to your frying pan.

4. Divide your egg mixture between two smaller-sized omelette pans and cook over a medium heat. Once your bottom layer of egg has solidified enough to hold its shape, flip the omelette to cook the other side.

5. Once your egg has been fully cooked, divide the filling between your 2 omelettes and add a scoop of your fresh salsa.

6. Serve!

Spinach, Goat Cheese, & Chorizo Omelette (Serves 2)

Ingredients:

4 Eggs

2 ounces of Crumbled Fresh Goat Cheese

4 ounces of Chorizo Sausage

1/2 tablespoon of Butter

2 cups of Baby Spinach Leaves

1 tablespoon of Water

Sliced Avocado (Optional)

1/4 cup of Salsa Verde (Optional)

Directions:

1. Remove the chorizo from its casing and fry in your medium-sized saute pan until fully cooked.

2. Beat your eggs and water in your small-sized bowl.

3. Take the chorizo out of the pan with your slotted spoon and set it to the side. Wipe your pan of any remaining grease with a clean paper towel.

4. Melt the butter in the same pan over a low heat. Add the beaten eggs to your pan, then put the chorizo, crumbled goat cheese, and spinach on half of the egg mixture. Cook on a low heat for around 3 minutes until slightly firm, then fold the empty side over the side with the filling on it.

5. Cover the pan with foil or your pot cover and leave on a low heat for another few minutes until the eggs are cooked through. If the bottom is browning too fast, turn off your stove and leave the pan covered for up to 10 minutes and the residual heat should "bake" it until the center has been cooked fully.

6. Add your avocado slices and salsa verde if so desired.

7. Serve!

Crab, Chili, & Herb Omelette (Serves 2)

<u>Ingredients:</u>

3 1/2 ounces of White Crab Meat

2 Eggs

1 Small Diced Red Chili

1 tablespoon of Chopped Dill

1 tablespoon of Chopped Coriander

1 tablespoon of Low-Fat Crème Fraîche

1 tablespoon of Chopped Chives

Olive Oil

Herb & Leaf Salad (Optional)

Chili Sauce (Optional)

Directions:

1. Mix together your crab, herbs, chili, and crème fraîche and season well.

2. Beat your eggs with some seasoning until pale. Heat 1 teaspoon of oil in your small-sized frying pan and pour in your eggs, making a thin omelette. When your omelette is set, tip your crab mixture in, fold in half and warm through for another minute.

3. Add your herb salad and chili sauce if so desired.

4. Serve!

Baked Eggs w/ Spinach (Serves 6)

<u>Ingredients:</u>

6 Small Eggs

17 1/2 ounces of Spinach

1 3/4 ounces of Sliced Mushrooms

1 Finely Diced Shallot

2 tablespoons of Low-Fat Crème Fraîche

1 clove of Crushed Garlic

2 tablespoons of Gruyère Cheese

2 teaspoons of Dijon Mustard

Olive Oil Spray

Toast (Optional)

<u>Directions:</u>

1. Heat your oven to 350 degrees. Heat your spray of olive oil in a pan and fry your shallot until soft.

2. Fry your mushrooms until the juice given off has evaporated and they turn golden. Add your garlic and fry for about minute. Add your spinach and stir until wilted. Add your crème fraîche and Dijon. Season well.

3. Place your mushrooms and spinach into a baking dish and spread out, making 6 dips in your mixture. Crack your eggs into the dips, sprinkle over your gruyere (avoiding the yolks). Bake for approximately 12 to 15 minutes until the whites have set and your yolks are cooked to your liking.

4. Add toast if so desired.

5. Serve!

Eggs & Bacon w/ A Twist (Serves 6)

Ingredients:

6 Hard-Cooked Organic Extra Large Eggs

1/4 teaspoon of Dried Organic Thyme

12 slices of Organic Bacon

3 1/2 ounces of Cream Cheese

Directions:

1. Preheat the oven to 400 degrees.

2. Prepare the cream cheese filling: Combine cream cheese and thyme in your small-sized bowl and mix with your spoon until mixed well. Cover and set to the side.

3. Peel the eggs and cut them lengthwise with your sharp knife.

4. Remove the yolks. Fill your 6 egg white halves with cream cheese filling. Cover with the remaining 6 egg white halves.

5. Take 2 bacon slices per filled egg and wrap the eggs tightly in the bacon slices.

6. Place the wrapped eggs in your shallow ceramic or glass baking dish and bake for around 30 minutes.

7. Remove from the oven.

8. Serve!

Squash Toast w/ Feta, Sumac & Poached Egg (Serves 1)

Ingredients:

3 1/2 ounces of Peeled Butternut Squash (Cut Into Small Cubes)

4 Quartered Cherry Tomatoes

1 Egg

1 teaspoon of Pomegranate Molasses

1 ounce of Crumbled Feta

1 teaspoon of White Wine Vinegar

1 slice of Toasted Rye Bread

Pinch of Sumac

Directions:

1. Put your squash in a microwavable container with 4 tablespoons of water, the molasses, and seasoning. Mix together well and cover tightly with cling film. Microwave on high for approximately 5 to 10 minutes until tender. Remove your cling film (be careful about any steam escaping). Allow it to cool for a few minutes. Drain off any water.

2. Add a pinch of sumac then mash with your fork.

3. Bring your small-sized deep pan of water to a gentle simmer and add your vinegar. Swirl the water in a circle, then crack your egg into the middle. Poach for around 2 to 3 minutes until the white is set but your yolk is runny. Drain your egg with a slotted spoon then dry it with a paper towel.

4. Mash your squash onto the toast, sprinkle with your feta, and add your tomatoes. Top with your egg, a pinch of sumac, and season.

5. Serve!

Smoked Haddock & Spinach Rye Toast (Serves 2)

Ingredients:

3/4 ounce of Smoked Haddock

3 Eggs (Room Temperature)

7 ounces of Baby Spinach

1 ounces of Finely Grated Pecorino Romano

3 1/2 ounces of Semi-Skimmed Milk

3 long slices of Toasted Rye Bread

Garlic Oil

Directions:

1. Bring your small-sized pan of water to a boil and gently lower in your eggs. Boil for approximately 7 minutes, then immediately scoop out of the pan and place into cold water for a couple minutes to cool. Peel and set to the side.

2. Put your haddock into a small-sized pan and pour over your milk. Top up with water if you need to, to cover the fish completely. Bring to a simmer and poach gently for 2 to 3 minutes until your fish is opaque and begins to look flaky.

3. Remove from your pan, discard the skin and any bones. Break into large chunks.

4. Blanch your spinach by pouring water over it, through a sieve, and squeeze out all the water using the back of your spoon. Place into your bowl, season, add 1 teaspoon of garlic oil and grated Pecorino.

5. Top your rye toasts with your spinach and add chunks of your haddock. Cut your eggs into quarters and add these. Season well with black pepper and scatter over the remaining cheese.

6. Serve!

Smashed Broad Beans On Toast (Serves 6)

<u>Ingredients:</u>

10 1/2 ounces of Broad Beans (Blanched & Double-Podded)

1 ounce of Pecorino

1 clove of Garlic

2 1/2 ounces of Extra-Virgin Olive Oil

1/2 Lemon (Tested & Juiced)

6 slices of Toasted Sourdough

Handful of Rocket

Pinch of Chili Flakes (Optional)

<u>Directions:</u>

1. In your food processor blitz 1/4 of the broad beans, all the rocket, garlic, Pecorino, lemon zest and juice with your olive oil and some seasoning.

2. Add your remaining broad beans and pulse a couple times to leave it chunky.

3. Spoon onto your toast, sprinkle with your chili flakes and drizzle with olive oil.

4. Serve!

Low-Carb Waffles (Serves 1)

<u>Ingredients:</u>

3 Egg Whites

1/2 teaspoon of Baking Powder

2 tablespoons of Coconut Flour

1 packet of Stevia

2 tablespoons of Unsweetened Almond Milk

<u>Directions:</u>

1. Whip 2 of your egg whites to stiff peaks.

2. Once you have stiff peaks, stir in the coconut flour, stevia, milk, sweetener, baking powder, and 1 egg white.

3. Heat up your waffle iron to the highest temperature, and grease or spray it with your nonstick spray. Pour in your batter.

4. Cook in your waffle iron until brown. Should take around 3 to 4 minutes. Remove and add any desired toppings.

5. Serve!

Low-Carb Cereal (Serves 15)

Ingredients:

1 cup of Sunflower Seeds

1 cup Unsweetened Flaked Coconut

1 cup of Pumpkin Seeds

1 cup of Sliced Almonds

2 teaspoons of Cinnamon

1/2 cup of Hemp Hearts

1/2 cup of Pecans

1/2 teaspoon of Vanilla Extract

1/4 teaspoon of Vanilla Stevia Drops

Directions:

1. In a large-sized bowl, stir together all of your ingredients until combined together well.

2. Lay out on a rimmed baking pan and bake at 350 degrees for around 7 to 8 minutes.

3. Allow it to cool. Store in an airtight container.

4. Serve!

Coconut Overnight Oats (Serves 6)

Ingredients:

21 ounces of Half-Fat Coconut Milk

10 1/2 ounces of Porridge Oats

1 tablespoon of Chia Seeds

1 tablespoons of Maple Syrup

1 tablespoons of Pumpkin Seeds

Pinch of Cinnamon

Toasted Coconut Flakes

Directions:

1. Put all your ingredients into a bowl. Mix well, cover with cling film and leave it overnight in your refrigerator.

2. Mix in more milk to serve if it's too stiff, spoon into bowls and top with your toasted coconut flakes.

3. Serve!

Coconut Flour Porridge Breakfast Cereal (Serves 1)

Ingredients:

2 tablespoons of Coconut Flour

1 Large Egg (Beaten)

2 teaspoons of Butter

2 tablespoons of Golden Flax Meal

1 tablespoon of Sukrin Gold

3/4 cup of Water

1 tablespoon of Heavy Cream

Salt

Directions:

1. Place coconut flour, salt, golden flax meal, and water into your small-sized pot over a medium-high heat. When it begins to simmer, turn it down to a medium and whisk until it begins to thicken.

2. Remove coconut flour porridge from the heat and add your beaten egg, little by little, while whisking continuously. Place back on the heat and continue to whisk until your porridge thickens.

3. Remove from the heat and continue to whisk for around 30 seconds before adding your cream, butter, and sweetener.

4. Garnish with your favorite toppings.

5. Serve!

Breakfast Cookies (Serves 8)

Ingredients:

1 Egg (Beaten)

1 3/4 ounces of Melted Butter

1 tablespoon of Maple Syrup

3 tablespoons of Soft Light Brown Sugar

3 1/2 ounces of Jumbo Porridge Oats

1 3/4 ounces of Wholemeal Flour

1 teaspoon of Baking Powder

1 3/4 ounces of Chopped Dates

1 3/4 ounces of Raisins

Pinch of Mixed Spice

Pinch of Ground Cinnamon

Directions:

1. Heat your oven to 350 degrees. Put your egg in a bowl with your melted butter, sugar and maple syrup. Mix the flour, baking powder, oats, dates, raisins, and spices. Pour the liquid ingredients into the dry. Mix together well until combined, then leave for approximately 10 minutes for the ingredients to meld.

2. Add large spoonfuls of your mix to a baking tray lined with baking paper and push down to flatten. Bake for approximately 15 to 17 minutes, or until risen, crisp and golden at the edges (the middle will stay quite soft). Leave to cool on your tray for approximately 10 minutes, then transfer to your wire rack to cool completely. Keep in an airtight container for up to 3 days.

3. Serve!

Breakfast Smoothie Bowl (Serves 4)

Ingredients:

14 ounces of Frozen Red Berries or Smoothie Mix

13 1/2 ounces of Almond Milk

1 Peeled Ripe Banana

4 tablespoons of Greek Yogurt

2 Pitted & Chopped Dates (Optional)

Chia, Pumpkin Seeds, or Hemp Seeds

Blueberries or Raspberries

Goji Berries

Desiccated Coconut

Oats or Granola

Bee Pollen

Directions:

1. Blend your frozen berries, banana, yogurt and half your milk in a blender until smooth.

2. Taste it. If it's not sweet enough, add your dates and blend again. It should be a thicker consistency than a normal smoothie but runny enough to pour.

3. Add more almond milk a little at a time to get a pourable smoothie, and divide between your small-sized bowls.

4. Top with as many toppings as desired.

5. Serve!

Two-Tone Freezer Smoothie (Serves 4)

Ingredients:

1 Large Sliced Banana (Can Freeze Ahead of Time)

1/2 Frozen Avocado

13 1/2 ounces of Apple Juice

1 Peeled & Chopped Kiwi Fruit

2 Handfuls of Fresh or Frozen Blueberries

1 Halved Lime

Handful of Baby Spinach

Ice

Directions:

1. Put half your avocado, half your banana, the spinach, kiwi fruit and half your apple juice in a blender. Add 3 cubes of ice and squeeze in a lime half. Blend until smooth then pour into your 4 glasses.

2. Rinse out your blender then add the rest of the avocado and banana, the blueberries, the rest of the apple juice, 3 more ice cubes and the juice of another half of lime, squeezed.

3. Blend until smooth. Pour over a spoon onto the top of your green smoothie so you have 2 layers.

4. Decorate with extra blueberries.

5. Serve!

Super Green Smoothie (Serves 1)

Ingredients:

1/4 Peeled & Chunked Cucumber

1/4 Peeled & Chunked Avocado

1 Large Juiced Kiwi Fruit

1 Juiced Lime

Handful of Young Spinach Leaves

Directions:

1. Put your cucumber, avocado, spinach, and fruit juices into a smoothie maker or blender and whiz until smooth.

2. Dilute with a splash of water if you desire.

3. Serve!

Chapter Six: The 5:2 Diet Lunch Recipes

In this chapter, I will share with you 10+ 5:2 diet lunch recipes you can easily make yourself. I'll include a few beginner recipes and a few recipes that are more advanced. These recipes are all under 600 calories per serving and will work on both your fasting days and non-fasting days. On fasting days you may want to stick to a 1/2 serving for each of your two meals otherwise you'll exceed your calorie allowance for the day.

BBQ Chicken Cobb Salad (Serves 4)

Ingredients:

Salad:

2 Boneless, Skinless Thin-Sliced Chicken Breasts

2 Large Eggs

6 cups of Chopped Romaine Lettuce

4 slices of Bacon (Diced)

3 tablespoons of BBQ Sauce

2 Roma Tomatoes (Diced)

1 Avocado (Halved, Seeded, Peeled & Diced)

1 cup of Canned Corn Kernels (Drained)

1 cup of Canned Black Beans (Drained & Rinsed)

Freshly Ground Black Pepper

Kosher Salt

Buttermilk Ranch Dressing:

1/4 cup of Plain Greek Yogurt

1/4 cup of Sour Cream

1/2 cup of Buttermilk

1/2 teaspoon of Dried Dill

1/4 teaspoon of Garlic Powder

1/2 teaspoon of Dried Parsley

Freshly Ground Black Pepper

Kosher Salt

Directions:

1. To make your buttermilk ranch dressing, whisk together your buttermilk, dill, Greek yogurt, sour cream, parsley, garlic powder, salt, and pepper in a small-sized bowl. Set to the side.

2. Heat your large-sized skillet over a medium high heat. Add the bacon and cook until brown and crispy. Should take around 6 to 8 minutes. Transfer to your paper towel-lined plate. Set to the side.

3. Season your chicken breasts with pepper and salt. Add to your skillet and cook, flipping once, until cooked through. Should take around 3 to 4 minutes per side. Allow it to cool before dicing into bite-size pieces.

4. In your medium-sized bowl, add your chicken and BBQ sauce. Gently toss to combine. Set to the side.

5. Place your eggs in a large-sized saucepan and cover with cold water by 1-inch. Bring to a boil and cook for around 1 minute. Cover your eggs with a tight-fitting lid and remove from the heat. Set to the side for around 8 to 10 minutes. Drain well and allow it to cool before peeling and dicing.

6. To assemble your salad, place your romaine lettuce in a large-sized bowl. Top with the arranged rows of bacon, eggs, BBQ chicken, tomatoes, avocado, beans, and corn.

7. Add the buttermilk ranch dressing as desired.

8. Serve!

Mushroom & Asparagus Salad (Serves 1)

Ingredients:

12 Asparagus Spears

8 Walnut Halves

8 Medium Chestnut Mushrooms

1 Spring Green Onion

1 teaspoon of Shaoxing Rice Wine

1 teaspoon of Soy Sauce

Handful of Fresh Coriander

Directions:

1. Rinse, trim, and chop the vegetables. Quarter your mushrooms, cut the asparagus into 3 to 4 pieces, and finely slice your spring onion.

2. In the frying pan, sauté your mushroom and asparagus over a medium heat.

3. Once the vegetables begin to soften, add your spring onion, soy sauce, and rice wine to your pan, and continue to sauté until your spring onions are cooked and the liquid has reduced.

4. Meanwhile, heat your separate frying pan to a high temperature, and toast your walnuts until they are golden brown and the oils are beginning to emerge.

5. Toss the walnuts together with the asparagus mixture. Add your fresh coriander.

6. Serve!

Courgetti Som Tam Salad (Serves 2)

Ingredients:

2 Courgettes

3 1/2 ounces of Green Beans (Cooked & Cut Into 8cm Pieces)

1 Shredded Carrot

3 1/2 ounces of Cherry Tomatoes (Halved)

1 tablespoon of Tamari

1 Juiced Lime

1 Finely Sliced Bird's Eye Chili

1 tablespoon of Soft Brown Sugar

Small Bunch of Torn Coriander

Small Bunch of Torn Mint

1 tablespoons of Chopped Roasted Peanuts

Directions:

1. Use your spiralizer to make long, thin courgette strands and add these to your bowl with your carrot and green beans.

2. Add your cherry tomatoes, tamari, lime juice, chili, and palm sugar to a mortar and mix and bash together with a pestle.

3. Pour over the courgette and mix well. Leave to marinate for approximately 15 minutes.

4. Add your torn coriander and mint to the courgettes and toss well.

5. Serve with a sprinkling of your chopped peanuts.

6. Serve!

Crispy Chickpea & Kale Caesar Salad (Serves 4)

Ingredients:

14 ounces of Chickpeas (Tin, Rinsed, & Drained)

3 1/2 ounces of Kale (Large Stalks Discarded)

1 teaspoon of Garlic Powder

1/2 clove of Crushed Garlic

2 tablespoons of Finely Grated Parmesan

1/2 Juiced Lemon

2 tablespoons of Red Wine Vinegar

2 tablespoons of Greek Yogurt

2 teaspoons of Olive Oil

1 Finely Sliced Red Onion

Olive Oil

Directions:

1. Heat your oven to 400 degrees. Make your pickled onions by pouring your vinegar over the onions, add a pinch of salt and leave to pickle while you make your salad.

2. Pat your chickpeas dry with kitchen paper. Toss with 1 teaspoon of oil, grated Parmesan, garlic powder, and season with lots of black pepper and a little salt. Put onto your shallow baking tray and cook for approximately 30 to 35 minutes until golden and crisp. Pace the kale into your large-sized bowl, add 1 tablespoon of lemon juice and massage your kale to soften the leaves a little.

3. To make your dressing mix all your ingredients with the remaining lemon juice and some seasoning. Add a little water to your dressing to make it pourable. Drizzle half into the kale and toss until all the leaves are coated. Divide between two plates and add your crisp chickpeas to the salad. Top with your pickled onions and the remaining dressing.

4. Serve!

Courgetti, Pea, & Artichoke Salad w/ Pistachio Pesto (Serves 2)

Ingredients:

2 Trimmed Courgettes

2 tablespoons Toasted Shelled Pistachios

3 1/2 ounces of Fresh or Defrosted Frozen Peas

1 clove of Crushed Garlic

1 Bunch of Basil (Leaves Picked)

1/2 Lemon (Zested & Juiced)

6 Sliced Artichoke Hearts (From A Jar)

Olive Oil

Salad Leaves

<u>**Directions:**</u>

1. Put half your pistachios, all the basil leaves, garlic, lemon juice and zest together and blend to a paste in your small blender. Add 1 teaspoon of oil and season. Loosen with more lemon juice or water if you need to, to make a pesto.

2. Put your courgettes through a spiralizer, or peel them into long, thin ribbons with a vegetable peeler, then cut into thin strips. Put them into your bowl with the peas, artichokes and salad leaves. Chop your remaining pistachios and add them to your bowl.

3. Pour over your pesto and toss with your salad.

4. Serve!

Vegan Fajita Bowl w/ Cauliflower Rice (Serves 2)

<u>Ingredients:</u>

1 Small Chopped Cauliflower

1 Large Red Pepper (Seeded & Sliced)

1 tablespoon of Chipotle Paste

1 Sliced Red Onion

7-ounce tin of Chopped Tomatoes

1/2 teaspoon of Garlic Salt

1/2 teaspoon of Cumin Seeds

1/2 teaspoon of Dried Oregano

1/2 teaspoon of Smoked Paprika

1/2 teaspoon of Chili Flakes

Olive Oil

Black Pepper

1/2 Small Sliced Avocado (Optional)

Lime Wedges (Optional)

Coriander Leaves (Optional)

<u>Directions:</u>

1. Heat 1 teaspoon of oil and fry your pepper and onion for approximately 10 minutes until soft and lightly golden. Add your chipotle paste, tomatoes and a splash of water. Simmer for approximately 15 to 20 minutes until your sauce has thickened a little bit.

2. For your spiced cauliflower rice, pulse your cauliflower in a food processor until it looks like grains. Toast your cumin in a non-stick frying pan in 1 teaspoon of olive oil, add your paprika, garlic salt, oregano, and chili flakes. Fry for approximately 1 minute before adding your cauliflower rice. Stir-fry for an additional 4 to 6 minutes until your cauliflower is tender, and smells a little toasted. Season well with some black pepper.

3. Divide between your bowls. Add your peppers on top, the avocado, and coriander leaves. Place lime wedges on the side to squeeze over your dish if so desired.

4. Serve

Szechuan Prawn Noodles (Serves 1)

Ingredients:

3 1/2 ounces of Raw Peeled King Prawns

1/4 teaspoon of Ground Szechuan

3 1/2 ounces of Cooked Fine Egg Noodles

1 clove of Crushed Garlic

1 Small Red Chili (Seeded & Diced)

1 teaspoon of Grated Ginger

1 Shredded Pak Choi

2 teaspoons of Soy Sauce

1 teaspoon of Rice Vinegar

4 Spring Onions (Trimmed & Sliced)

Groundnut Oil

Directions:

1. Heat 1 teaspoon of oil in a wok and add your ground Szechuan pepper, ginger, garlic, and chili. Stir-fry for a couple minutes until fragrant.

2. Add your pak choi, 3 of your spring onions and the prawns. Cook for approximately 2 to 3 minutes until your prawns are pink.

3. Add your noodles and toss to reheat. Add your soy sauce and vinegar and cook for 1 minute until your prawns are cooked completely through and your noodles are hot.

4. Sprinkle with your remaining spring onion.

5. Serve!

Chicken Mole (Serves 4)

<u>Ingredients:</u>

6 Skinless Chicken Thighs (Cut Into Strips)

2 Red Onions (1 Chopped & 1 Sliced Into Rings)

16 ounces of Chicken Stock

2 cloves of Crushed Garlic

1/4 block of Willie's Mexican Mole Cacao

14-ounce tin of Chopped Tomatoes

Pinch of Chili Powder

Small Bunch of Coriander Leaves

Olive Oil

Cooked Rice (Optional)

Lime Wedges (Optional)

Directions:

1. Cook your chopped onion and garlic in 1 tablespoon of olive oil until softened. Add your chicken and fry for approximately 2 minutes, then stir in your tomatoes and stock and bring to a simmer.

2. Add your mole cacao and chili and cook for another 30 minutes, until thickened.

3. Stir in half your coriander and add rice, more coriander, onion rings, and lime wedges.

4. Serve!

Chicken & Asparagus Lemon Stir Fry (Serves 4)

<u>Ingredients:</u>

1 1/2 pounds of Skinless Chicken Breast (Cut Into 1-Inch Cubes)

2 tablespoons of Reduced-Sodium Soy Sauce

1/2 cup of Reduced-Sodium Chicken Broth

1 tablespoon of Canola Oil

2 teaspoons of Cornstarch

2 tablespoons of Water

6 cloves of Chopped Garlic

1 bunch of Asparagus (Ends Trimmed & Cut Into 2-Inch Pieces)

1 tablespoon of Fresh Ginger

3 tablespoons of Fresh Lemon Juice

Fresh Black Pepper

Kosher Salt

<u>**Directions:**</u>

1. Lightly season the chicken with salt. In a small-sized bowl, combine the chicken broth and soy sauce. In a second small-sized bowl combine your cornstarch and water and mix together well to combine.

2. Heat your large-sized non-stick wok over a medium-high heat, when hot add 1 teaspoon of your oil, then add your asparagus and cook until tender-crisp. Should take around 3 to 4 minutes. Add your garlic and ginger and cook until golden. Should take around 1 minute. Set to the side.

3. Increase your heat to high and add 1 teaspoon of oil and half of the chicken. Cook until browned and cooked through. Should take around 4 minutes on each side. Remove and set to the side and repeat with your remaining oil and chicken. Set to the side.

4. Add the soy sauce mixture; bring to a boil and cook for about 1 1/2 minutes. Add your lemon juice and cornstarch mixture and stir well. When it simmers return the chicken and asparagus to your wok and mix well. Remove from the heat.

5. Serve!

Asian Chicken Burgers w/ Pickled Red Cabbage (Serves 4)

<u>Ingredients:</u>

4 Chopped Skinless Chicken Breasts

1/2 Small Red Cabbage (Finely Shredded)

4 tablespoons of Panko Breadcrumbs

1 Juiced Lime

1 tablespoon of Chopped Ginger

3 tablespoons of Rice Vinegar

1/2 stalk of Lemongrass (Finely Shredded)

2 tablespoons of Sriracha Chili Sauce

1 teaspoon of Sesame Oil

1 teaspoon of Soy Sauce

Small Bunch of Coriander (Finely Chopped)

Round Lettuce Leaves

<u>Directions:</u>

1. Toss your cabbage with your lime juice and vinegar and season. Put to one side at room temperature until you're ready to serve. Heat your oven to 450 degrees.

2. Blitz your chicken, coriander, ginger, and lemongrass quickly in your blender until combined. Mix in your sesame oil, panko, sriracha and season with soy sauce.

3. Mold into 4 burgers. Put onto your lined baking tray and transfer to your oven. Cook for approximately 15 minutes on each side until golden and cooked through.

4. Place on lettuce leaves. Top with your pickled cabbage and add more sriracha on the side.

5. Serve!

Griddled Tuna w/ Olive & Parsley Salad (Serves 2)

Ingredients:

2 Tuna Steaks

1 Finely Chopped Shallot

15 Pitted Green Olives (Quartered)

1 teaspoon of Capers

1/2 bunch of Chopped Parsley Leaves

1 Zested & Juiced Lemon

Olive Oil

Black Pepper

Salt

Cooked New Potatoes

<u>Directions:</u>

1. Rub your tuna steaks with olive oil and season well.

2. Fry or grill for approximately 1 to 2 minutes on each side.

3. Mix your olives with the shallot, lemon zest, capers, and parsley. Season well and dress with your lemon juice and some olive oil.

4. Plate with your tuna steak and potatoes.

5. Serve!

Portobello & Halloumi Burgers (Serves 2)

<u>Ingredients:</u>

4 Portobello Mushroom Caps w/ Stems Removed

2 Thick Slices of Tomato

2 tablespoons of Olive Oil

2 Thin Slices of Halloumi Cheese

3 1/2 tablespoons of Balsamic Vinegar

1 handful of Basil Leaves

Pepper

Sea Salt

<u>Directions:</u>

1. Heat your grill to a medium-high heat (about 450 degrees). Wash your mushroom caps and dry. In a shallow bowl, combine your balsamic vinegar and olive oil. Place your mushrooms grill side down in the mixture.

2. Once the grill is hot, grill your mushrooms on the grill side first for around 5 minutes or until they start to sweat. Flip and grill around 2 to 3 minutes more. Add your halloumi to the grill and grill for 2 minutes on each side over a relatively high heat until grill marks form on the cheese and it becomes soft and pliable. Sprinkle your salt and pepper onto the tomato.

3. Assemble your "burger" with your mushroom as the bun, the halloumi cheese as the burger, the lightly salted tomato, and fresh basil leaves.

4. Serve!

Blackened Fish Sandwich w/ Smoked Paprika Mayo (Serves 4)

Ingredients:

Blackened Fish:

4 Firm White Fish Fillets

1 teaspoon of Smoked Paprika

1 teaspoon of Golden Caster Sugar

1 teaspoon of Garlic Salt

1/2 teaspoon of Finely Ground Celery Seed

1 teaspoon of Onion Salt (Optional)

Smoked Paprika Mayo:

5 tablespoons of Mayonnaise

1 teaspoon of Smoked Paprika

1/2 clove of Crushed Garlic

1 Zested Lime

Black Pepper

Serving:

4 Large Soft Buns

4 Small Lettuce Leaves

1 Medium Thinly Sliced Red Onion

1 Large Sliced Beefsteak Tomato

Directions:

1. Mix your mayonnaise, lime zest, garlic, and smoked paprika in your small-sized bowl. Crack some black pepper in and stir.

2. For your fish, mix your spices and sugar then sprinkle this over all sides of your fish so that it's covered completely.

3. Heat your barbecue or griddle pan. Grill your fish on direct heat for approximately 2 to 3 minutes on each side depending on the thickness.

4. Spread a spoonful of your mayonnaise on the bottom half of each bun. Add your lettuce, tomatoes, and onions and a piece of fish. Top with the other half of your bun.

5. Serve!

Spaghetti Squash

Ingredients:

1 Spaghetti Squash

1 1/2 cups of Cooked Chickpeas

3/4 cup of Toasted Hazelnuts

3 cloves of Garlic

1 bunch of Kale

Pinch of Crushed Chilies

Pecorino Romano (Hard Sheep's Milk Cheese)

Olive Oil

Sea Salt

Directions:

1. Preheat the oven to 400 degrees.

2. Prepare the spaghetti squash by cutting it in half lengthwise, removing your seeds, rubbing the inside of each half with a drizzle of olive oil, then seasoning with the salt and pepper. Place face down on a lined baking tray and place in your oven. Cook for around 45 minutes.

3. While the squash is baking, prepare the rest of your filling. Wash your kale well and remove the tough center rib of each leaf. Roughly chop the kale into small-sized pieces.

4. Heat the ghee, oil, or butter in your frying pan, then add your minced garlic, crushed chilies to taste, along with a pinch of sea salt. Cook for about 2 minutes until fragrant, then add your chopped kale and cook until the leaves are bright green and just beginning to lose structure. Throw in the chickpeas and cook until warm. Remove from the heat.

5. Remove the squash from the oven when it is cooked through. Using your fork, scrape out all the insides, which will pull away from the shell in strands, like spaghetti. Place all the strands in your bowl and toss with your kale and chickpea mixture. At this point, you can either serve it from the bowl or mix everything together and place back in one-half of the empty squash shells for a nicer presentation. Sprinkle with chopped toasted hazelnuts and shaved Pecorino Romano.

6. Serve!

Chapter Seven: The 5:2 Diet Dinner Recipes

In this chapter, I will share with you 15+ 5:2 diet dinner recipes you can easily make yourself. I'll include a few beginner recipes and a few recipes that are more advanced. These recipes are all under 600 calories per serving and will work on both your fasting days and non-fasting days. On fasting days you may want to stick to a 1/2 serving for each of your two meals otherwise you'll exceed your calorie allowance for the day.

Tofu Steak w/ Beetroot Noodles & Dukkah (Serves 1)

Ingredients:

5 1/4 ounces of Firm Tofu (Patted Dry)

1 Large Peeled Beetroot

1 tablespoon of Finely Chopped Flat-Leaf Parsley

1 tablespoon of Finely Chopped Chives

1 tablespoon of Finely Chopped Mint

1 Zested & Juiced Clementine

Olive Oil

Salt

Green Salad

Dukkah:

1 tablespoon of Chopped Blanched Hazelnuts

1 teaspoon of Cumin Seeds

1 teaspoon of Coriander Seeds

1/2 teaspoon of Black Peppercorns

1/4 teaspoon of Dried Mint

1/4 teaspoon of Fennel Seeds

Sea Salt

Directions:

1. Season your tofu with salt, press between pieces of kitchen paper and put a heavy chopping board on top to draw some of the water out.

2. To make your dukkah, toast the nuts and spices (except the mint) in a dry frying pan for a few minutes until fragrant. Roughly blitz until coarsely ground in a spice grinder. Mix in your dried mint and a pinch of sea salt.

3. Spiralize your beetroot or use a julienne peeler to make 'noodles'. Heat your grill to high. Brush 1 teaspoon of olive oil over your tofu and grill for a few minutes on both sides, until it has a golden crust. Scatter over 2 teaspoons of the dukkah and grill again for a few minutes.

4. Mix your herbs, zested and juiced clementine, a pinch more dukkah and toss with your beetroot noodles. Add a tiny drizzle of olive oil and top with your tofu steak.

5. Serve!

Aubergine Steaks w/ Sesame Dressing & Pomegranate (Serves 2)

Ingredients:

1 Large Aubergine (Cut Into 4 Thick Slices Lengthwise)

2 teaspoons of Za'atar

1 tablespoon of Pomegranate Molasses

1 teaspoon of Tahini

1 tablespoon of Olive Oil

2 teaspoons of Fat-Free Yogurt

1/2 Juiced Lemon

1 teaspoon of Toasted Sesame Seeds

1 1/2 ounces of Lighter Feta

Bunch of Coriander (Leaves Torn Off)

Handful of Salad Leaves

Directions:

1. Heat your griddle pan or grill to hot. Mix your olive oil, za'atar, and some seasoning. Brush mixture over your aubergine steaks on both sides.

2. Char your aubergine slices for approximately 6 to 8 minutes on each side until they become soft all the way through (they shouldn't feel spongy if you cut one with a knife).

3. Keep your cooked aubergine covered with foil to steam and keep warm while you cook your remaining slices.

4. Whisk your tahini, lemon juice, yogurt, and half your seeds with a little water until you can drizzle it. Toss your coriander with the salad leaves.

5. Lay your za'atar aubergine steaks onto plates, crumble over your feta, drizzle with the sesame dressing and pomegranate molasses, and scatter over the remaining sesame seeds. Add a coriander salad on the side.

6. Serve!

Tandoori Lamb Steaks w/ Chili-Spiked Slaw (Serves 4)

<u>Ingredients:</u>

4 Lamb Leg Steaks (Trimmed of All Fat)

1 clove of Crushed Garlic

2 Seeded & Finely Diced Red Chili

1 Small Piece of Ginger (Peeled & Grated)

1 tablespoon of Tandoori Masala Spice Mix

1/2 teaspoon of Ground Cumin

1/2 teaspoon of Ground Turmeric

3 1/2 ounces + 4 tablespoons of Fat-Free Yogurt

2 Peeled & Shredded Carrots

1 Finely Sliced Red Pepper

2 Shredded Spring Onions

1/4 Finely Sliced Red Cabbage

2 teaspoons of Groundnut Oil

1 Juiced & Zested Lemon

Handful of Chopped Mint Leaves

Directions:

1. Make your marinade for the lamb by mixing together your garlic, spices, ginger, 3 1/2 ounces of yogurt, half your lemon juice, and some seasoning.

2. Pour over your lamb steaks and rub in well. Cover and chill for at least 2 hours or overnight if you can.

3. To make your slaw, toss all your remaining ingredients together with some seasoning and a good squeeze of the remaining lemon. Mix the 4 tablespoons of yogurt with the mint, a little lemon zest, and season.

4. Heat your griddle pan or grill to hot. Remove your steaks from the marinade, letting any excess drip off. Char your lamb for approximately 4 minutes on each side, or longer if you like.

5. On the side, add your chili slaw and mint yogurt.

6. Serve!

Tuscan Pork Steaks (Serves 3)

<u>Ingredients:</u>

3 Pork Loin Steaks (Trimmed of All Fat)

6 Chopped Plum Tomatoes

2 cloves of Crushed Garlic

14-ounce tin of Butterbeans (Rinsed & Drained)

1 tablespoon of Balsamic Vinegar

5 1/4 ounces of Kale

1 tablespoons of Small Capers

1/2 Zested & Juiced Lemon

Handful of Chopped Oregano

Handful of Chopped Basil

Olive Oil Spray

__Directions:__

1. Heat a spray of olive oil in your frying pan and fry half your garlic for 1 minute. Add your tomatoes, vinegar, a splash of water, lemon zest, and capers. Simmer for approximately 2 to 3 minutes, to soften. Leave to cool.

2. In another pan, fry your remaining garlic in a spray of olive oil. Add your kale, butterbeans, and the lemon juice with a splash of water, if you need to, to wilt your kale. Season well.

3. Season your pork chops and spray with a little olive oil. Grill your pork chops for approximately 2 to 4 minutes on each side until cooked through. Add your oregano and basil to the tomatoes and season. Divide your kale and beans between 3 plates or bowls. Top with your pork steaks and the tomato relish.

4. Serve!

Lamb Koftas w/ Kale Salad (Serves 4)

<u>Ingredients:</u>

14 ounces of Minced Lean Lamb

2 teaspoons of Ground Cumin

2 teaspoons of Cayenne Pepper

1/2 Finely Diced Red Onion

1/2 Zested & Juiced Lemon

2 tablespoons of Chopped Mint

2 tablespoons of Chopped Parsley

3 1/2 ounces of Brussels Sprouts

3 1/4 ounces of Low Fat Natural Yogurt

7 ounces of Kale (Tough Stalk Removed & Leaves Shredded)

Oil

Flatbreads

Directions:

1. Mix your minced lamb, red onion, 1 teaspoon of cumin and cayenne, lemon zest, and herbs. Season and form into 12 small-sized sausages. Chill for at least 1 hour.

2. Mix your yogurt with 1 teaspoon of cumin and half your lemon juice. Blanch your sprouts for approximately 6 minutes. Add your kale for the last 3 minutes. Drain well.

3. Shred your sprouts, add your kale and toss with 1 teaspoon of oil, the remaining lemon juice, and an extra pinch of cayenne.

4. Grill the koftas, turning, for 10 minutes until cooked through.

5. On the side, add your salad, yogurt, and flatbreads.

6. Serve!

Moroccan Vegetable & Chickpea Tagine (Serves 4)

<u>Ingredients:</u>

1 Chopped Red Onion

2 cloves of Chopped Garlic

14-ounce tin of Chickpeas (Rinsed & Drained)

1/2 teaspoon of Ground Cumin

1/2 teaspoon of Ground Cinnamon

1/2 teaspoon of Ground Coriander

1 Chopped Aubergine

1 Red Pepper (Seeded & Chopped)

4 Chopped Vine Tomatoes

1 Chopped Courgette

2 tablespoons of Harissa

8 1/2 ounces of Vegetable Stock

4 Prunes (Pitted & Sliced)

Olive Oil Spray

Chopped Flat-Leaf Parsley

Steamed Couscous (Optional)

Directions:

1. Fry your onion and garlic in a spray of olive oil for approximately 5 minutes. Add your spices and fry for around 1 minute until fragrant. Add the vegetables and fry for approximately 8 to 10 minutes until they're coated in the spices and start to take on some color.

2. Add your chickpeas, stock, prunes, and harissa. Season and simmer for approximately 15 to 20 minutes until your vegetables are tender.

3. Scatter over your parsley and add couscous.

4. Serve!

One-Pot Chicken w/ Cannellini Beans & Chorizo (Serves 4)

Ingredients:

4 Whole Chicken Thighs

3 1/2 ounces of Light Chicken Stock

1 Red Onion (Cut Into Slim Wedges)

1 tin of Cannellini Beans (Rinsed & Drained)

1/2 teaspoon of Chopped Rosemary

Small Chunk of Diced Chorizo

Olive Oil

Directions:

1. Heat your oven to 400 degrees.

2. Put your chicken thighs in an oiled baking dish or roasting tin, tucking your onions underneath the thighs. Season well. Pour light chicken stock or water in the bottom. Roast for approximately 30 minutes, then add your chorizo and cook for another 15 minutes.

3. Add your beans and rosemary and stir everything together (including your onions). Roast for approximately 10 minutes.

4. Serve!

Chicken Piccata (Serves 2)

<u>Ingredients:</u>

2 Skinless Chicken Breasts

6 3/4 ounces of Chicken Stock

2 tablespoons of Rinsed Capers

1 Lemon (1/2 Zested & Juiced - 1/2 Sliced)

1 clove of Crushed Garlic

1/2 Bunch of Chopped Flat-Leaf Parsley

Olive Oil

Green Salad

Cauliflower Rice

<u>Directions:</u>

1. Cut your chicken breasts through the middle lengthwise, to open them out like a book. Put them between 2 pieces of cling film and bash them with a rolling pin to 1cm thick.

2. Heat 1 teaspoon of oil in a frying pan. Fry your flattened chicken breasts for approximately 4 minutes on each side until golden and cooked through. Remove from your pan. Season and leave to rest under foil.

3. Add your capers and garlic and fry for a minute, then add your lemon juice, zest, and stock. Simmer for a few minutes until the sauce thickens slightly. Add the chicken back to the pan, with the lemon slices and parsley and spoon over the sauce.

4. On the side, add your green salad and cauliflower rice.

5. Serve!

Chicken & Parmesan Fennel (Serves 8)

Ingredients:

3 1/2 ounces of Chicken Breast (Cut It Length-Ways)

7 ounces of Fennel (Cut Into Eighths)

5 ounces of Boiled Potatoes

1 tablespoon of Greek Yogurt

1 teaspoon of Walnut Oil

2 teaspoons of Grated Parmesan

1/4 teaspoon of Smoked Paprika

1 tablespoon of Roughly Chopped Parsley

Directions:

1. Rub the chicken with half the oil and season well with salt, pepper, and smoked paprika.

2. Preheat the oven to 390 degrees. Lay your fennel in a roasting tin with the chicken and sprinkle carefully with your Parmesan, making sure as little as possible falls in the tin. Bake for around 10 to 15 minutes, until browned, and the chicken is cooked through but not dried out.

3. Slice your chicken breast. Mix the last 1/2 teaspoon of walnut oil with the Greek yogurt, adding plenty of seasoning and a teaspoonful or so of water to make a thick pouring consistency.

4. Top with parsley.

5. Serve!

Chicken w/ Agrodolce Sauce (Serves 2)

Ingredients:

2 Skinless Chicken Breasts

1 Red Onion (Halved & Thinly Sliced)

3 1/2 ounces of Halved Cherry Tomatoes

3 stalks of Thinly Sliced Celery

1/2 teaspoon of Sugar

1 tablespoon of Red Wine Vinegar

1 tablespoon of Seasoned Flour

Small Handful of Chopped Flat-Leaf Parsley

Olive Oil

Watercress

<u>Directions:</u>

1. Slice your chicken breasts in half horizontally so that you have 4 thin pieces. Cover with your baking paper and flatten gently with a rolling pin or the bottom of a heavy pan. Dust with your seasoned flour, shaking off any excess.

2. Heat 1 tablespoon of olive oil in a non-stick frying pan and brown your chicken well on both sides. Remove then cook your onion and celery in the same pan for 3 minutes and season. Add your tomatoes and cook for approximately 3 to 4 minutes until they start to break down. Add your vinegar and sugar. Put your chicken back in the pan and cook for approximately 3 to 4 minutes until cooked through then stir in your parsley.

3. On the side add your green salad.

4. Serve!

Beef Bourguignon (Serves 6)

<u>Ingredients:</u>

16 ounces of Extra-Lean Diced Braising Steak

13 1/2 ounces of Beef Stock

18 Peeled Shallots

3 tablespoons of Seasoned Plain Flour

4 Peeled & Diced Carrots

17 ounces of Red Wine

9 ounces of Halved Chestnut Mushrooms

2 Bay Leaves

2 sprigs of Thyme

2 tablespoons of Chopped Flat-Leaf Parsley

Olive Oil

<u>Directions:</u>

1. Heat your oven to 325 degrees.

2. Sprinkle your flour over the beef and toss well.

3. Heat 1 tablespoon of oil in a large-sized casserole dish and fry your beef in batches until browned. Drain on kitchen paper.

4. Add your onions, carrots, and mushrooms to your oil and fry for approximately 10 minutes until the onions are turning golden and the carrots have softened.

5. Add a splash of wine and stir to loosen the crispy bits at the bottom of your pan, before adding the drained beef pieces, the stock, herbs and the rest of the wine.

6. Put on a tight-fitting lid with a layer of tin foil underneath the lid. Cook for approximately 2 hours until the beef is tender and add seasoning if needed.

7. Remove your meat and vegetables with a slotted spoon. Simmer the sauce on the hob to reduce and thicken it.

8. Return the meat and vegetables to your pan and gently reheat. Scatter over the parsley.

9. Serve!

Lentil Meatballs w/ Fresh Tomato Sauce (Serves 4)

<u>Ingredients:</u>

7 ounces of Brown Lentils

3 1/2 ounces of Finely Chopped Mushrooms

1 Diced Onion

6 Large Diced Vine Tomatoes

1 clove of Crushed Garlic

4 tablespoons of Porridge Oats

1 Zested Lemon

Green Salad

Tomato Sauce

Olive Oil Spray

Small Handful of Basil

Cooked Orzo (Optional)

Directions:

1. Heat your oven to 400 degrees. Rinse your lentils well, then simmer in boiling water for approximately 15 minutes until starting to go soft. Fry your onion in a spray of oil until soft but not brown. Allow it to cool.

2. Drain your lentils well and put in a blender with your cooled onion, mushrooms, oats and lemon zest. Pulse until the mix is combined (but don't blend to a mush). Season, and roll into 16 balls, then put them on a lined baking sheet. Bake for approximately 30 minutes until golden and firm, turning them halfway through.

3. Meanwhile, make the tomato sauce by frying your garlic in a spray of olive oil for 1 minute before adding your tomatoes with a splash of water. Simmer for around 5 minutes, until the tomatoes start to break down. Cook the orzo and drain well.

4. Season your tomato sauce and stir in the basil. Add your balls to the orzo in shallow bowls, add the tomato sauce, and add the green salad on the side.

5. Serve!

Black Bean & Corn Fajitas (Serves 2)

<u>Ingredients:</u>

10 ounces of Black Beans (Cooked & Drained)

6 ounces of Sweetcorn

2 tablespoons of Olive Oil

1 Large Onion

4 tablespoons of Fajita Spice Mix

1 Zucchini

1 Red Bell Pepper

8 Tortilla Wraps

Thick Sour Cream

Salsa

<u>**Directions:**</u>

1. Slice your zucchini, red pepper, and onion into thin strips.

2. Heat your oil in your large-sized frying pan and add your vegetables and spices.

3. Stir fry until your vegetables are soft and coated in the spice mixture. Add your black beans and corn and cook over a medium heat until warmed through.

4. Gently warm your tortillas.

5. Add sour cream, salsa, and a crunchy salad on the side.

6. Serve!

Egg Fried Rice (Serves 2)

Ingredients:

2 Eggs

6 ounces of Basmati Rice

4 Spring Onions (Green Onions / Scallions)

1 tablespoon of Vegetable Oil

4 ounces of Peas

Directions:

1. Cook the rice according to the packet instructions. Leave in your saucepan, away from the heat.

2. Heat the oil in a large-sized frying pan, and fry your eggs. Flip your eggs to fry the second side. (You're aiming for over medium consistency, and it doesn't matter if the yolks get broken.)

3. Chop your egg into small-sized pieces.

4. Add your rice and stir into the egg.

5. Slice the spring onions and add along with your peas.

6. Stir fry for a couple of minutes.

7. Serve!

Smoked Salmon Pitta Pizza (Serves 1)

Ingredients:

1 ounce of Smoked Salmon Slices

1 White Pitta Bread

1 teaspoon of Drained Capers

1 tablespoon of Low Fat Cream Cheese Chive and Onion

1 1/2 ounces of Lettuce Leaves

1/4 Red Onion (Peeled & Finely Diced)

1 Lemon Wedge

Fresh or Dried Dill

Directions:

1. Preheat the oven to 350 degrees.

2. Spread your pitta bread with your low-fat cream cheese then top with your smoked salmon pieces. Scatter the red onion over the top and then the capers.

3. Bake for approximately 10 minutes, or until your pitta bread is golden and crispy around the edges.

4. Add your lemon wedge and fresh chopped dill as well as some fresh lettuce leaves.

5. Serve!

Creole Cod (Serves 4)

Ingredients:

4 6-ounce Cod Fillets (About 1-Inch Thick)

1/2 teaspoon of Creole Seasoning Blend

2 teaspoons of Dijon Mustard

2 teaspoons of Olive Oil

1/2 teaspoon of Salt

1 tablespoon of Fresh Lemon Juice

Chopped Fresh Parsley

Cooking Spray

Directions:

1. Preheat the oven to 400 degrees.

2. Combine your first mustard, creole, salt, and oil. Brush evenly over fish.

3. Place your fish on a foil-lined baking sheet coated with cooking spray. Bake at 400 degrees for approximately 17 minutes or until the fish flakes easily when tested with a fork. Drizzle juice evenly over fish. Garnish with parsley, if desired.

4. Serve it up!

Chapter Eight: The 5:2 Diet Soups, Sides, & Snacks Recipes

In this chapter, I will share with you 10+ 5:2 diet soups, sides and snacks recipes you can easily make yourself. I'll include a few beginner recipes and a few recipes that are more advanced. These recipes are all under 600 calories per serving and will work on both your fasting days and non-fasting days. On fasting days you may want to stick to a 1/2 serving for each of your two meals otherwise you'll exceed your calorie allowance for the day.

Mexican Quinoa Stuffed Peppers (Serves 3)

<u>Ingredients:</u>

6 Bell Peppers

5 ounces of Cherry Tomatoes

9 ounces of Cooked Quinoa (1 packet)

1 Small Red Onion

2 teaspoons of Olive Oil

1 tablespoon of Diced Jalapeños

5 ounces of Sweetcorn

2 tablespoons of Fresh Coriander

Juice of 1 Lime

1 3/4 ounces of Grated Cheese (Optional)

<u>**Directions:**</u>

1. Preheat the oven to 400 degrees.

2. Wash your peppers, cut the tops off with a sharp knife and scoop out the seeds.

3. Rub the outside of your peppers with olive oil and arrange on your baking tray.

4. Finely dice your red onion and quarter the cherry tomatoes.

5. Mix the onion, sweetcorn, tomatoes, quinoa, coriander, lime juice, jalapeños, and cheese (if using) in a large-sized bowl.

6. Fill your peppers with your quinoa mixture and replace the pepper tops.

7. Bake for around 25 to 30 minutes, until your pepper skins are starting to blacken.

8. Serve!

Quick Quinoa & Black Bean Vegan Chili (Serves 4)

<u>Ingredients:</u>

7 ounces of Quinoa (Rinsed & Drained)

1 Chopped Onion

13 1/2 ounces of Chopped Tomatoes

2 cloves of Crushed Garlic

1 Chopped Red Chili

2 teaspoons of Ground Cumin

13 1/2-ounce tin of Black Beans (Rinsed & Drained)

1 teaspoon of Hot Smoked Paprika

1/2 teaspoon of Chili Powder (Optional)

20 ounces of Vegetable Stock

1 Small Sliced Avocado

Olive Oil Spray

Coriander Leaves

<u>Directions:</u>

1. Fry your onion, garlic, and red chili in a spray of olive oil until soft, then add your spices, including the chili powder if you want it spicy.

2. Add your quinoa, stock, tomatoes, and black beans. Season well. Cover and simmer for approximately 30 minutes until your quinoa is tender and the sauce has thickened.

3. Top with avocado slices and coriander leaves.

4. Serve!

Red & White Quinoa Bowl (Serves 2)

<u>Ingredients:</u>

7 ounces of Mushrooms

1 1/2 ounces of Red Quinoa

2 ounces of White Quinoa

2 Red Pointed Peppers

1 tablespoon of Wholegrain Mustard

1 tablespoon of Lemon Juice

<u>Directions:</u>

1. Cook the quinoa according to the instructions on the packet.

2. Chop your peppers into large-sized chunks and quarter your mushrooms.

3. Mix the lemon juice and mustard together.

4. Add your vegetables and the lemon/mustard to a frying pan. Saute over a medium heat for around 5 minutes until softened.

5. Add your quinoa to the pan with the vegetables and toss through to coat in the lemon dressing.

6. Serve!

Smoked Salmon Chowder (Serves 8)

<u>Ingredients:</u>

1 pound of Potatoes (Peeled & Cubed)

8 ounces of Smoked Salmon (Cut Into 1/2-Inch Pieces)

2 tablespoons of Butter

1/2 cup of All-Purpose Flour

2 cloves of Chopped Garlic

1 tablespoon of Olive Oil

1 cup of Chopped Onion

1/2 teaspoon of Paprika

1 teaspoon of Dried Tarragon

1/2 cup of Chopped Celery

6 cups of Chicken Broth

1/4 teaspoon of Hot Sauce

1 tablespoon of Fresh Lemon Juice

1 teaspoon of Dried Dill Weed

1 cup Half and Half

1 teaspoon of Dried Thyme

1/4 cup of White Wine

1 teaspoon of Ground Black Pepper

1 teaspoon of Salt

<u>Directions:</u>

1. In a large-sized stock pot over a medium-high heat, combine your butter, onion, olive oil, garlic, and celery. Cook approximately 8 to 10 minutes, or until your onions are transparent. Sprinkle flour over the mixture and stir well to make a dry roux. Gradually add your chicken broth and stir until slightly thickened. Stir in your potatoes, dill, thyme, tarragon, and paprika. Reduce heat to a medium, cover, and simmer for approximately 15 minutes.

2. Stir in the salmon, wine, lemon juice, hot sauce, pepper, and salt. Simmer over a low heat, uncovered for approximately 10 minutes.

3. Mix in your half-and-half and continue to simmer for around 30 minutes, stirring occasionally. Do not let your chowder boil after adding the half-and-half.

4. Serve!

Butternut & Sage Risotto (Serves 4)

Ingredients:

7 ounces of Arborio Rice

1 Small Chopped Onion

27 ounces of Hot Vegetable Stock

9 ounces of Butternut Squash (Peeled & Diced)

2 tablespoons of Grated Parmesan

Chopped Sage Leaves

Olive Oil

Directions:

1. Fry your onion gently in 1 tablespoon of oil in a deep frying pan or sauté pan until soft but not browned. Add your squash and rice and stir for a few seconds to coat the grains with oil.

2. Add a couple of ladles of stock and bring to a simmer. Cook, stirring, until almost all the stock is absorbed.

3. Add the rest of the stock a little at a time, cooking until each addition is absorbed before adding the next until your squash is soft and the rice is creamy but still al dente. Stir in your sage and season well.

4. Divide your risotto between bowls and sprinkle with cheese.

5. Serve!

Pork Fillet w/ Pepper Stew (Serves 4)

Ingredients:

14-ounce Pork Tenderloin

2 Large Red Peppers (Seeded & Sliced)

7 ounces of Chicken Stock

1 Sliced Red Onion

1 tablespoon of Red Wine Vinegar

2 sprigs of Thyme

2 cloves of Sliced Garlic

1 teaspoon of Smoked Paprika

Olive Oil

Chopped Flat-Leaf Parsley

Directions:

1. Trim your tenderloin of all fat and sinew. Cut into 12 medallions.

2. Put your pork pieces between two pieces of cling film and bash them so they are about 1cm thick. Season both sides.

3. Heat 1 teaspoon of oil in your non-stick frying pan, and fry the pork for approximately 2 minutes on both sides, until golden and cooked through.

4. Scoop out of your pan, then stir-fry your peppers, garlic, and onions in another teaspoon of oil for approximately 5 minutes. Add the stock and the thyme sprigs.

5. Add a lid or a sheet of baking paper and simmer for approximately 10 to 15 minutes until your peppers are soft.

6. Add your vinegar and paprika and season. Fry for around 2 minutes with your lid off, stir in the pork pieces (with any resting juices) to warm in the stew for a minute.

7. Scatter with parsley.

8. Serve!

Prawn & Mushroom Miso Soup (Serves 1)

Ingredients:

1 3/4 ounces of Cooked Peeled Prawns

2 tablespoons of Miso Soup Paste

4 Sliced Shiitake Mushrooms

1 3/4 ounces of Pak Choy (Leaves Separated)

1 teaspoon of Soy Sauce

1 ounce of Soba Noodles (Soaked In Boiling Water For 2 Minutes & Drain)

1 tablespoon of Chopped Coriander (Optional)

1/2 Sliced Red Chili (Optional)

Directions:

1. Mix your miso paste with 17 ounces of boiling water and bring to a simmer. Add your mushrooms and greens. Simmer for approximately 4 minutes until softened. Add your prawns to warm through for 1 minute, then remove from the heat.

2. Add your noodles, season with soy, then scatter with the coriander and chili.

3. Serve!

Fiery Chickpea & Harissa Soup (Serves 4)

Ingredients:

1 Chopped Onion

14-ounce tin of Chickpeas (Drained)

2 stalks of Diced Celery

2 Diced Carrots

1/2 teaspoon of Ground Cumin

2 tablespoons of Tomato Purée

2 tablespoons of Harissa

25 ounces of Vegetable Stock

Olive Oil

Handful of Chopped Parsley Leaves

Directions:

1. Cook your onion in 1 tablespoon of olive oil until softened. Add your carrot and celery and cook for approximately 5 minutes. Stir in your cumin and harissa and cook for a minute.

2. Add the rest of your ingredients, season and bring to a simmer. Cook for approximately 15 minutes then stir in your parsley.

3. Serve!

Thai Mushroom Soup (Serves 4)

Ingredients:

9 ounces of Field Mushrooms

2 Large Onions

7 ounces of Chestnut Mushrooms

6 Large Garlic Cloves

3 1/2 ounces of Baby Button Mushrooms

1 teaspoon of Toasted Sesame Oil

1 tablespoon of Tomato Puree

1 3/4 ounces of Coconut Cream

1 Small Red Chili

3/4 ounce of Fresh Chopped Cilantro

2 tablespoons of Red Thai Curry Paste

2 pints of Boiling Water

Fresh Ginger (1-Inch)

Directions:

1. Finely chop the onions and field mushrooms. Fry in your sesame oil for about 10 minutes until soft.

2. Chop your ginger, garlic, and chili. Stir into the onion/mushroom mixture and fry for a few more minutes.

3. Add your curry paste, tomato puree, and around 1/2 pint of boiling water. Simmer over a low heat for approximately 45 minutes.

4. Dissolve the coconut cream into your soup and add the rest of your boiling water.

5. Trim your button mushrooms and cut the chestnut mushrooms into thick slices. Add these to the soup, along with your chopped cilantro. Simmer for another 5 minutes until all your mushrooms are tender.

6. Stir the cilantro through just before serving, and reserve a little to garnish.

7. Serve!

Mushroom Miso Soup (Serves 1)

<u>Ingredients:</u>

4 Small Chestnut Mushrooms

2 Spring Onions (Scallions /Green Onions)

2 cups of Mushroom Stock

3 1/2 ounces of Tofu

1 tablespoon of Miso Paste

<u>Directions:</u>

1. Heat up the mushroom stock and dissolve it in your miso paste.

2. Chop up the mushrooms and tofu into small bite-sized pieces and slice the spring onions.

3. Add your vegetables and tofu to your broth and simmer for approximately 5 minutes until heated through.

4. Serve!

Vegetarian Puttanesca Sauce (Serves 2)

Ingredients:

20 Large Kalamata Olives

1 1/2 cups of Tomato Sauce

3 tablespoons of Olive Oil

1 Large Onion

2 cloves of Garlic

1 tablespoon of Capers

Cooked Pasta

Directions:

1. Chop the onion and crush your garlic.

2. Heat your oil in a large-sized frying pan and fry the onion and garlic until soft.

3. Add the tomato sauce, capers, and olives. Simmer for around 15 to 20 minutes to infuse the flavors.

4. Add sauce over your pasta.

5. Serve!

Spiced Cauliflower (Serves 2)

Ingredients:

21 ounces of Cauliflower

1/2 Red Pepper

5 1/4 ounces of Chestnut Mushrooms

1/2 teaspoon of Turmeric

7 ounces of Vegetable Stock

3 1/2 ounces of Cherry Tomatoes

1 Small Onion

1 teaspoon of Sunflower Oil

2 teaspoons of Garam Masala

4 cloves of Garlic

4 Cardamom Pods

Directions:

1. Cut your cauliflower into florets. Roughly chop the onion, pepper, and mushrooms. Cut your tomatoes in half. Finely dice your garlic.

2. Heat the oil in a large-sized saucepan.

3. Fry the onion, pepper, and garlic until the onions are soft.

4. Add your spices and mushrooms and fry for a couple more minutes.

5. Add the vegetable stock and cauliflower florets. Simmer for approximately 10 minutes over a medium heat, turning regularly to coat all the cauliflower florets in the spiced stock.

6. Add the tomatoes, cover, and simmer gently for another few minutes to soften your tomatoes.

7. Use a slotted spoon to leave behind any excess liquid.

8. Serve!

Conclusion

Thanks for reading my book. I hope this guide on the 5:2 diet has provided you with all the necessary information you needed to get going. Don't put off getting started. The sooner you begin, the sooner you'll start to notice a positive progression in your overall health and well-being. While the results may vary from person to person, they will eventually come if you stick to the 5:2 diet information you discovered in this book.

If you still have any unanswered questions I suggest checking out one of the apps, books, or resource sites I shared earlier. When I first got started on the 5:2 diet these sites had many of the answers I was searching for. They were truly an invaluable resource to have at my fingertips. I steadfastly believe in always trying to expand one's base of knowledge. I highly recommend you check out some of the books I suggested as they are all filled with wonderful information.

Good luck. I wish you nothing but the best!